The Early Life of Jeomie East

Struggling with Sickle Cell Anemia

By

Phyllis East

ISBN: 0-7596-6801-9

1stBooks - rev. 3/28/02

Introduction

by

Editor

and

The Early Life of

Jeomie East

Struggling With Sickle Cell Anemia

9/15/96

THE EARLY LIFE OF JEOMIE EAST

The introduction of Jeomie East into the world began with her birth on March 23, 1966 in Bellevue Hospital in New York. Her parents, Phyllis East and Robert East Jr. lived in a high rise apartment on 34th Street in Manhattan, New York. Jeomie was the first born of four children, with two other sisters named Weomie and Neomie, and a brother Robert East III. Jeomie's mother had no complications during her pregnancy nor any at the time of the delivery of Jeomie. A healthy 6 pounds 8 ounce baby girl, she brought much joy to her parents.

Nearly every mother catalogs the ages of growth and development of their child. Experiencing the normal activities associated with childhood, Jeomie began crawling at the age of 6 months. By 10 months, she pulled herself up to a table to walk around it.

No complications nor signs of the disease were discovered until her visit with the doctor for her immunization shots. The lab testing accidently discovered traces of sickle cell in Jeomie's blood. The family doctor explained the disease to Jeomie's parents,

Phyllis and Robert. They were unaware that they were carriers of the trait which caused the disease in Jeomie. Their sorrow was intensified as they learned from the doctor the complications which Jeomie would experience. Early death stole the life of many African American children. Phyllis and Robert would now be alerted to watch for behaviorial changes in Jeomie. Constant surveillance of Jeomie would occupy the thoughts of her parents.

Jeomie continued to engage in normal activity in her preschool years, showing signs of perception and awareness of the world around her. In elementary school,

Jeomie's parents learned that she was a very gifted child. Placed in the Intelligent Gifted Children (IGC) classes, she loved learning and earned the distinction of being listed on the school honor roll. Her second born sister Weomie, who also had the sickle cell anemia trait, attended the IGC classes too.

Jeomie refused to have it revealed that she had the disease sickle cell anemia. Wishing to be normal, Jeomie wanted no one to pity her. Possessing a beautiful poetic mind, she spent countless hours writing memorable lines of verse. Being kind and considerate besides intelligent, Jeomie had many friends who shared her love of learning.

As Jeomie grew older, she became more independent. Her mother Phyllis had often dressed Weomie and Jeomie alike. Some people even thought they were twins. Although she still loved her sister, dressing like Weomie did not interest her anymore.

Eventually, Jeomie began experiencing the sickle cell crisis, they became more frequent when she was older. Jeomie's mother would leave her work to stay with Jeomie in the hospital. Jeomie did not feel like herself during the sickle cell crisis. She wrote bold notes on colored construction paper stating to her sister Weomie that she wanted her to stay out of her personal belongings, the signs in the room would say:

STAY OUT THIS MEANS YOU

DON'T TOUCH

KEEP OFF PROPERTY

Jeomie kept these signs hanging on bedroom walls constantly. She knew her sister Weomie loved to sneak into her room and borrow her clothes, her digital games, and sometimes read her diary.

During the summer when school was out, Jeomie loved spending time with her brother Robert. He was seven years younger and had no traces of the disease or the trait. Other days she would go to the park with her sister Weomie to play kickball and run with the neighborhood children. She enjoyed riding her bicycle and fishing with the family in a little pond for crowdads.

When the third baby girl was born, Jeomie begged her father not to name the baby with a name ending in "eomie". Jeomie thought that since she was 17 years older than the baby, she would be able to convince her parents to name her sister a different name. Her father told to her that it was too late to change the baby's name. Neomie was loved and cherished by Jeomie, who spent hours playing outside in the backyard with her stuffed animals and her ball.

The evening hours were a special time for Jeomie. She appreciated the hours before bed because her favorite scientific and mystery movies were aired. At that time, she specifically wanted her sisters and brother to be quiet, not saying a word.

Jeomie was especially gifted in artistic activities. She enjoyed creating different animals by hand from yarn. It was her decision to take the yarn animals with her to the hospital so she could sell them to the staff. That made her time at the hospital a little more pleasant. Stuffed with cotton, the various animals almost came alive in their assorted forms. Beautiful dolls, soft teddy bears, fluffy cats, funny dogs, wild giraffes, sleek polar bears and smooth elephants covered the floor of Jeomie's hospital room.

Back at home, Jeomie's room exhibited an assortment of awards hanging on the wall: best creative worker, diplomas from school, best writer, and some others signifying her many achievements as a very talented individual. She like to keep her night light on before she went to sleep. As her mother watched her grow from newborn to teenager, she was inspired by Jeomie to live life to the fullest, with courage and bravery. Jeomie truly was a fine example for others to follow.

Biography

of

Jeomie East

9/3/96

Phyllis East

These past two years, my health has been the worst that I have lived through yet. The most difficult years for me concerning my health were 1981-82. Even with the amazing amount of trouble that I have endured, I always managed to pull through. I would like to give thanks to those who encouraged me to be strong and determined to fight my illness that I had encountered during these past few years. My disease is Sickle Cell Anemia, a disease where the blood cannot carry enough oxygen. The sickle cells die quickly and leave the body without enough red blood cells to supply the needed oxygen. The hemoglobin in sickle cells releases too much oxygen and if oxygen is reduced enough, the cells will be sickled.

Sickle Cell Anemia is an incurable disease, but can be controlled. A Sickle Cell Crisis occurs when a large number of sickle cells are present. They tend to pile up and stick together in the blood vessels. This makes it difficult or impossible for the blood to circulate. The illness often caused drastically reduced circulation and oxygen shortages, especially in the hands, feet, and bones. When this happens, prompt medical attention is required. During the crisis which is most painful, I am given oxygen, I-Vs, transfusions, and pain medication.

Sickle Cell Anemia is a life-threatening disease. It has caused the following problems:

Carditis and heart failure interfers with the heart pumping blood throughout the body.

Attythmia is a condition where the heart beats are irregular. Skipping and pounding heart beat is usually a sign of this.

Lupus S. L. E. is a disease that causes good blood cells to fight against the body, destroying its immune system.

Neurphytis occurs when the kidneys fail to work, causing internal problems. I have to take medication for this, otherwise I would go on for days without using the bathroom, as I experienced in earlier years.

Rheumatoid Arthritis causes the joints to be very painful and sometimes it becomes so painful that it is impossible to walk.

My spleen has been destroyed from the illness. It just sits in my body rotting away.

I am taking a total of 98 pills a week for all of these illnesses. The list follows:

Digoxin: 0.125 Mg. 1. (x) This is to slow my heart down just a little and it also strengthens the heart.

Folic Acid: 1 Mg. 1. This is an iron pill mainly for the Sickle Cell Anemia.

Erythromycin: 250 Mg. 1. this is used to help prevent infections.

Plaguenil: 200 Mg. 1. This is used to prevent lupus flare-ups.

Lasix: 20 Mg. 2 (x) This is used to get rid of extra fluid that could build up around the heart, making it difficult to breathe.

Theragram: 1. Really, this is just a vitamin.

Lorcainide: A 100 Mg. 3. (x) An experimental drug used to control irregular heart beats.

Aldactone: 25 Mg. 4. (x) This helps control blood pressure.

(See notation at end of chapter.)

My illness started again after a very long five years of remission. On September 9, 1981, I went to a neighborhood hospital room. The reoccurence of my problem caused my kidneys to hurt severely. Lupus was suspected and I had to have a kidney biopsy. That meant that a medical device was to be inserted into my kidneys to remove a piece of tissue. This procedure would be done at another hospital in the area. The doctor said that I was too ill to be moved to the second hospital. I remained 9 days at the first hospital, from September 9th to the 17th.

On the 20th of September, I entered the second hospital where I met a Kidney Specialist who performed my biopsy. It was very uncomfortable and the anaesthesia that they gave me did not put me to sleep. I felt everything; it was painful, but by then I was use to pain so I shed no tears. Later I learned that the doctor would be my permanent doctor. I remained in the hospital from September 20th to the 27th.

All went well up until the 16th of October. My hands were swollen and the cause was unknown. My next hospital visit was a long and impatient one for me. I wanted to go home for Halloween but was refused when I asked permission from the resident. We had Halloween at the hospital, but it just was not the same without my sister and brother.

Soon I had a roommate who was age 16. She had Lupus too and was a diabetic. We spent a very long time together. I found her quiet nice but quiet. I stayed in the hospital for 20 days from October 16th to November 3rd.

Not long after I returned home, I was once again readmitted at the second hospital for another Sickle Cell Crisis. Both arms hurt and ached. There I met a new doctor who was a Cardiac Specialist. My visit lasted 5 days from November 29th to December 3rd. I was happy to be able to be with my family again.

December was a cold month but I was determined not to get sick. Christmas was approaching and I had developed a bad cough. As each day witnessed my cold worsening, my body ached as I longed for some relief from the pain. I would cry silently by myself so not to worry my mother or cause her to become upset.

Phyllis East

By Christmas Eve I was so ill that I was moved to the emergency room which I had visited so many times before. I believed that the hospital staff would not keep me there long. The only real problem was that I could not catch my breath because of my continuous coughing. They listened to my lungs and privately called my doctor and heart specialist. Both physicians arrived to look at my x-rays. There was no doubt; they were going to admit me. I could not believe my sad Christmas Eve.

I had pneumonia and I did not even know it. I had to get treatment every 4 hours from a respiratory therapist who would pound on my back which felt very painful. Christmas went especially nice when my family brought my presents to me. I got everything I wanted, so did my sister and brother.

During this time at the hospital, I was advised to get a tutor. I also met another student who was 12 years old. He was a boy whom I had recognized from my school. He was one of the guards who I would talk to while waiting for my brother to come out of school. It was funny meeting him in the hospital over the holidays. He had heart trouble like I did but he looked healthy to me.

When New Years arrived on January 1, 1982, I was still stranded in the hospital. It was okay because I knew that I would be able to go home soon, which I did on January 4th. My last visit lasted 12 days from December 24th - January 4th of 1982, a very traumatic year for me.

At home I was lonely because I could not go to school, but I was being tutored at home to continue my education. School was very important to me. I did not wish to fall behind my classmates who were continuing to learn each in school.

February went well. Soon March came and I knew that this was going to be a good month because we had 3 birthdays in that month. My brother's birthday was on the 3rd, my sister's was on the 19th, and my birthday was on the 23rd. I was going to be 16.

March 11th was a school day for me because I was tutored. I was not feeling well. Later that day, I had another Sickle Cell crisis but I was use to the severe pain and I knew sooner or later the pain would ease up. Instead of relief from my pain, my suffering became intense and unbearable. My mother thought that it was the same as before, a mild crisis, so she was not in a rush to call my father. He was at work which was a thirty minute drive away from our home.

While I waited for the crisis to leave, I started to cry aloud, louder and louder. I had never felt so much pain in my entire life. My whole body was in so much pain that I could hardly stand the suffering. My joints were weakening, little by little; I was a mess. The only wish I had was that someone would cut off my arms and legs. Soon after that thought, my legs gave out. I could not walk or balance myself but most of all, I could not sit still.

My brother and sister watched me carefully to make sure that I would not role off the chair, while my mother quickly dialed my father to come to take me to the emergency center. He was unable to come. He was the only person working in the store and he told my mom that it was just impossible to close up the shop. My sister was terribly upset, and I was just delirious. Soon afterward, my mother called a friend who carried me to the car, and then drove me to the hospital which was 5 minutes away.

Into the emergency room we went with my mother hurriedly thanking the friend for the ride. We did not have to wait to sign any papers. They let us right through. That surprised me. Usually a person could be bleeding to death, and they insist that papers are signed before entry. We went right on through the opened automatic door where a nurse was there waiting to help me.

The very first thing they did was give me a I. V. and pain medication. After a while the pain eased to where I could tolerate it. At home when I went into a crisis, my tolerance of pain was excellent. It takes a lot to make me cry. One can imagine that a Sickle Cell crisis was a terrible experience. The nurses sent me upstairs after I had calmed down a little. I had oxygen in the tank, because I was barely getting any air on my own. Upstairs I felt better.

That night the family came to see me and I enjoyed their company. The next morning I called my tutor, and told him not to come to my house because I was not going to be there. I told him I was in the hospital. Later on that day he came to visit. I was feeling quite ill, and while he was there, my mother phoned me. I cried over the phone, telling her that my arms and legs still hurt. Soon he left, disappointed.

For the next few days I went downhill, not able to walk nor eat, and every movement was torture. That night the severe pain came back. I was crying, asking someone to help me. Soon a nurse did. I was getting uncontrollable, which caused just about all the nurses of that station to sit with me to calm me down.

After midnight my oxygen was not helping me even though I had it on. It was not enough. I was sweating up a storm. My clothes were soaked. That night was just awful. Sleep eluded me. Laying in bed just looking at the walls, I waited for the next pain medication. My suffering grew worse into the morning; I could barely open my eyes. Extremely weak from pain, my heart beat very fast. The doctors called my parents to tell them that I was going into intensive care. There were only six beds there in one very large room: I felt relieved that several nurses cared for us.

The nurses immediately hooked me up to a heart machine, then to the oxygen. They started more I.V.s, placing two in each arm. By then my veins had collapsed, so they had to cut my skin in order to insert the I.V.s. It was necessary for my bed to be in a sitting position to prevent me from gasping for air, even with the oxygen on. One of my I.V.s contained Lasix to help me to use the bathroom because my kidneys failed to function.

Several doctors examined me to decide what was to be done. Each day I was not permitted to eat or drink. Once in a while they would give me ice chips to prevent the heart from overworking. The days went slowly; I was experiencing heart failure. I could feel my self losing weight each day that they weighed me. If I lost weight, my heart would not have to work so hard. Eighty-eight pounds was quite a distance from one hundred ten pounds. I could see my ribs without any trouble. Often I contemplated during the days at the hospital; some days were good and some were bad, but in any cases, I would always give thanks.

I was assigned to an individual nurse. She never left my side during that shift. It was the 18th of March, one day before my sister's 15th birthday. Birthdays were very important to me. I felt sad that I was not going to be there to share it with her. The nurses offered me some comfort in my loneliness.

Later while I was watching television, I began to notice that my head was feeling tight, as if someone was tying a scarf around my head and pulling it tighter and tighter at each end. The pain just came out of nowhere, when suddenly I heard the alarm of my heart monitor. I passed out before the doctors and nurses arrived with the emergency kit.

When I opened my eyes, one doctor asked me my name. "Do you know where you are?", he asked. I went blank; I could not answer because I did not know. Subsequently, I was told that I had experienced a seizure. The alarm sounded to alert the hospital staff that my heart was in trouble.

When I heard this I was stunned. That night they took x-rays and E.K.G.s of my heart to determine what damage had occurred. The doctors discussed the situation and agreed that a cardiac catheterization was necessary. My heart specialist catheterized my upper thigh. He numbered me and cut my skin with a razor. I felt some discomfort, but not much. Then he inserted a long, thin wire that could reach the heart directly. I never knew why it was done, but I was glad when he took it out.

March 23rd arrived, and I was 16 at last. On this day they decided to move out of the unit and on to the floor. This was a last minute decision because someone needed the bed more than I did. It was the student I mentioned earlier, remember? He had a heart transplant. His results were unexpected. He died. Everyone was sad, and so was I. Some even cried. I did not. I was just surprised that he was only 12.

Although I was moved from intensive care, the hospital staff had me hooked up to everything. After a very lengthy recovery, I finally went home on April 9th, Good Friday. I had been in the hospital for 30 days from March 11th to April 9th.

A few days later on April 16th, I was readmitted for heart trouble. I was told that I had arrhythmia, irregular heart beats. If it was not controlled, I could go into heart failure. Once again the doctor warned us. On the 22nd of April, I found myself in the Cardiac care unit. The doctors talked my situation over and decided to try me on an experimental drug. They had my mother sign the papers of warnings of side-effects. The new drug worked. I left the hospital May 6th after remaining 22 days since April 16th.

I returned for a short time on May 22nd to I.C.U. for observation. My medicine level needed to be increased. I left on the 31st of May, Memorial day, after 10 days at the hospital. Summer had arrived. June went well and so did July. By the 12th of August I was hospitalized because I needed oxygen for shortness of breath. I left on the 20th after seven days.

September and October gave me no trouble. On Thanksgiving Day, November 25th, I went into the emergency room continuously vomitting. The reason was never found. My stomach ached. When I was able to keep down food, I was sent home on December 3. I had been at the hospital for over a week.

I thought that I was in the clear, but it was not four days before I was readmitted to the clinic by my heart specialist for arrhythmia. He requested that the hospital staff check my medication. I was having knee pain, a mild Sickle Cell crisis. I asked for pain medicine but the pain became worse. Once again I could not walk. I was in deep pain. They tried giving me a new pain medicine which was not addictive. It was called Talwen.

I continued sweating up a storm, vomitted from nausea, and hurt all over. The doctor ordered a transfusion. My dizziness almost prevented me from walking to the bathroom. When I was in the bathroom, I felt very dizzy, so I think I pushed the nurse button. The nurses found me on the floor trembling. They got me into the wheel chair that was in my room at the time and got me to bed. I was in bad shape.

The doctor thought that I had a Sickle Cell crisis of the brain which caused me to blackout. Then a nurse watched me all night. After I became worse, the Talwen was discontinued. They decided to give my a shot of Demoral. It made my head spin and it did nothing to ease my pain. I felt like I was losing my mind.

Later I progressed and felt good enough to go home on Christmas Eve. I could not believe that I had spent so much time in the hospital again. A new perspective on life had entered my thoughts. The past 17 days from December 8th through the 24th made me realize that I would not enjoy life as I had previously.

Various thoughts entered my mind as the holidays progressed. The New Year is coming soon, my health may improve in 1983. With the New Year, I would like to keep some thoughts in mind. A day of worry is more exhausting than a week of work. The longest day has had an end. Take care of the minutes and the hours will take care of themselves. In this world, it is not what we take up but what we give up, that makes us rich. Happiness is not having what one wants, but wanting what one has. People see your action, but God sees your motives.

Phyllis East

What is easy is seldom excellent, please all and no one will be pleased. Love all, trust few, do wrong to no one. Each morning look back upon the work of yesterday and then try to improve it. Whenever I can, I always try to help the next person. Life has a purpose, whether one choses to do wrong or right it will always come back in one way or another. No matter now long I live I will always keep this thought in mind. It is not how long one lives; it is what is accomplished while alive.

Jeomie East

December 25, 1982

Age 16

Closing Comment

by

Editor

and

Family Photos

9/15/96

Phyllis East

An autobiography is an intimate portrayal of the experiences and circumstances of one's life. The individual who wrote the short biography on the pages that follow was a respected, intelligent and enterprising young woman. She had acquired the wisdom necessary to ascertain a philosophy of life which is stated at the end of her story. The culture from which she drew her convictions and her strength is the African American tradition.

Hard work, intellectual convictions spiritual fortitude, self-respect, and a pragmatic awareness of life in the United States characterizes Jeomie. One becomes painfully aware of the meager housing which often shelters the African American family when viewing the photos of Jeomie East, and her family, and her relatives in the various settings.

Despite living in a racist Jeomie East was a honor student. a leader, and a director of ideas which influenced school classmates and teachers alike. After Jeomie passed away, a former teacher named Ms. Long asked permission of Jeomie's parents if she could establish a special writing award of two hundred dollars in the number of Jeomie East. Because Jeomie had been an excellent writer, Ms. Long wished to remember the memory of Jeomie East and her exceptional qualities. The letter from Ms. Long is dated April 3, 1990 and is included after the autobiography.

Phyllis East

JEOMIE EAST ESSAY CONTEST

DUE: April 27 (Fri.), 1990

STUDENTS   ELIGIBLE: MINORITY
SENIORS

QUESTION: IF YOU HAD A FATAL
DISEASE WHICH WOULD YOU
TAKE YOUR LIFE IN TEN YEARS,
HOW WOULD YOU LIVE YOUR
LAST DECADE ON EARTH?

WHAT WOULD YOU DO FOR
OTHERS? WHAT THREE THINGS OR

MORE WOULD YOU TRY TO ACCOMPLISH BEFORE YOU DIE? (I am going to read a sample of her philosophy of life from her writings at Awards Day as I present the $200.00 to the winner.)

LENGTH: 500 words or less

FORM: Typed (Double-Spaced)

PRIZE: $200.00 (Given at Awards Day)

JUDGING CRITERIA: Content, Grammar, Neatness, Originality

CONTEST DIRECTOR: Ms. Long rm. 203

JUDGES: Three English teachers who will not know your identity as you will be given an entry number.

Phyllis East

𝕵
𝕰
𝕺
𝔐
𝕵
𝕰

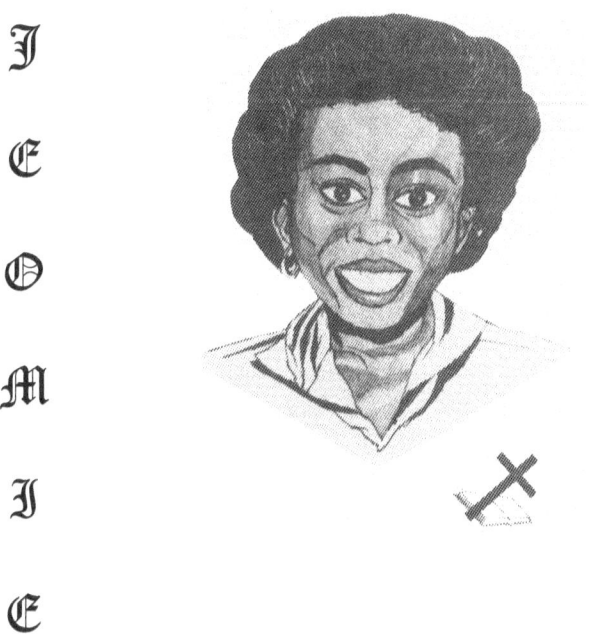

Elegy for Jeomie

by Ms. Long

For 3½ years, Room 203 was
your domain,

Where you courageously hid
your deepest pain.

Hr. 9 says you haunt the room

And sometimes that thought fills
them with gloom,

But I tell them that's just <u>not</u>
right,

For, Jeomie, you are <u>still</u> here as
our "Guiding Light!"

In loving memory of a special senior who
was close and dear to many...Jeomie East.

She had the inner strength to smile and care about others while she hid the pain she contained in- side.

She was like sunshine on a cloudy day. Whenever she came around, she seemed to be able to lift our spirits.

Although it's sad that Jeomie has left us, we can rest assured that the Lord has prepared a bet- ter peace for her. So instead of tears of sadness, cry tears of gladness.

By Lisa A. Hester

and

Christine M. Dixon

Phyllis East

"Whenever I can, I try to help the next person's life have a purpose. Whether you choose to do wrong or right, it will always come back to you in one way or another. No matter how long I live, I will always keep this thought in mind: it is not how long you live, but what you accomplish while you live, what is easy is seldom excellent, please all and you will please no one. Love all, trust few, do wrong to no one. Each morning look back upon your work of yesterday and then try to beat it."

Jeomie East
died January 19, 1984

Phyllis East

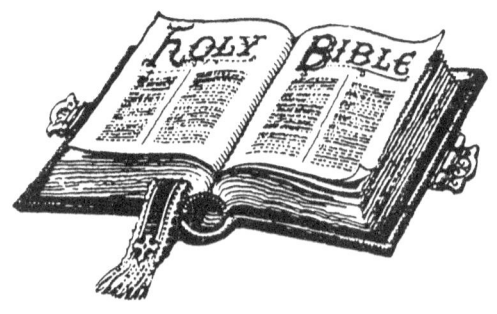

A Poem for Jeomie East

Jeomie's smile was silent as the

night.

Her memory will always be held

tight.

she was very talented, especially

in art.

All of her work really touched our
hearts.

She always stuck up for what was
right.

She looked to God as her guiding
light.

She was very quiet in her own
special way.

Maybe that's because she didn't
have much to say.

Words were insignificant whenever
she was near.

Our feelings overflowed, but never

in tears, over loss of tender

years.

by Terri dotson, Vincent Rudolph,

Kim Knight and Steve Modarai.

Phyllis East

Jeomie East

by Sherry Bowen

Jeomie, truth and of all honors,

She's paid the price of this war

down here.

In the heavens she will be so far

away.

Many battles she had fought

Fought with pain and winning by a

hair.

And yet not deserving the things

she met

Bearing the pain in silent tears,

She never said in her lifetime,

She'd soon go away.

She sleeps now with the ease of

pain.

Family Photos

Page 1

Some photos of Jeomie, her family, and some relatives have been included for the reader to appreciate the close and caring family life which Jeomie experienced. As exhibited by the photos, Jeomie was a beautiful African American infant who grew to become a darling little girl, and later a honor student who wrote poetry and philosophized about life. Dying from the complications of sickle cell anemia, her short life expressed a williness to face whatever path was before her.

What follows is a description of the photos as described by Weomie, Jeomie's sister who still remembers vividly the wonderful times that they experienced as sisters. Also included is a snapshot of one of Jeomie's yarn dolls, the kind which she sold during some of her weeks at the hospital. The yarn doll and yarn animals are among the treasures that her family holds dear in remembrance of their talented sister.

The photos following the last page are numbered 1-11.

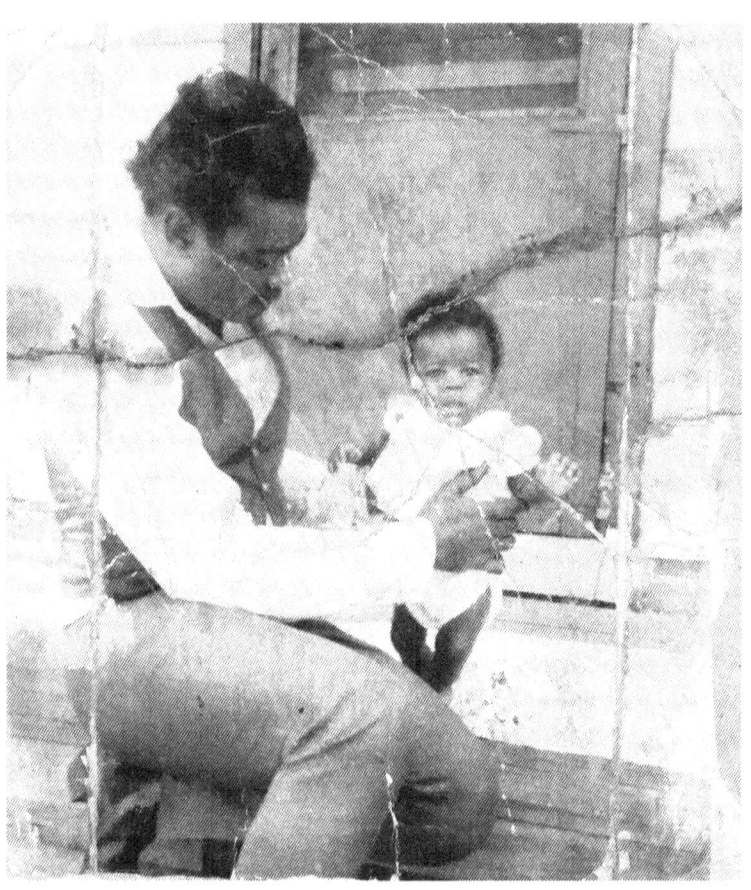

1. Jeomie's father Robert East is very proud to be holding her when she is 4 months at a relative's home in Baltimore Maryland.

Phyllis East

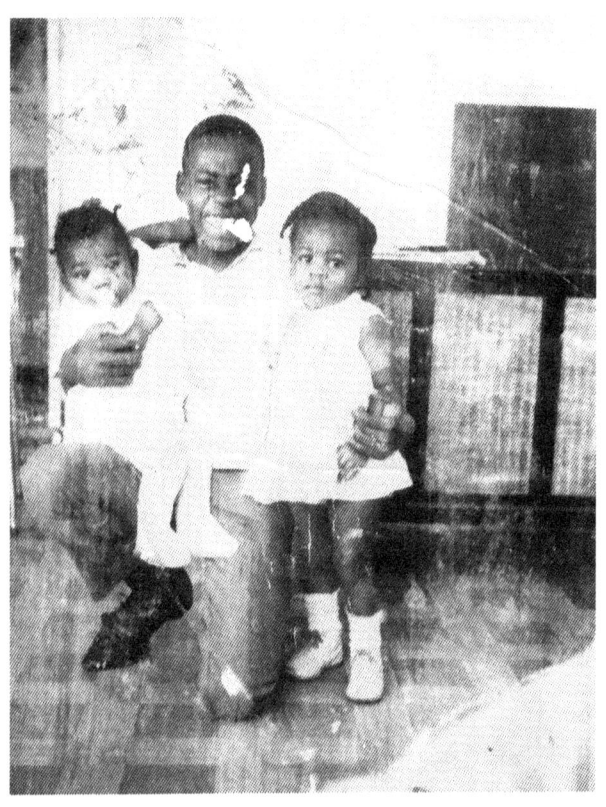

2. 2 year old Jeomie and 1 year old Weomie is sitting on their uncle's lap in Baltimore, Maryland.

Phyllis East

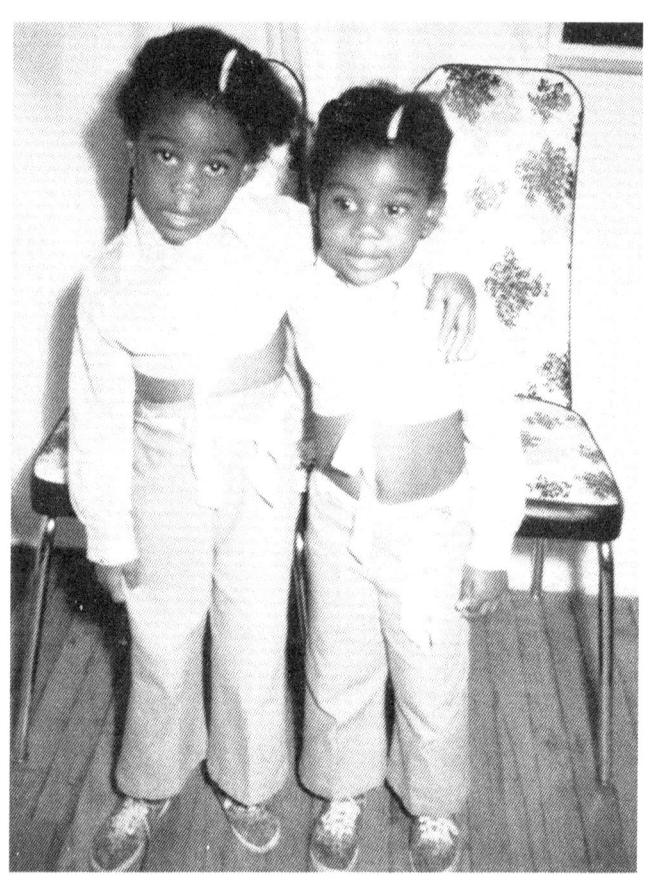

3. Looking like two African American princesses. Jeomie standing on the left is holding her sister Weomie.

Phyllis East

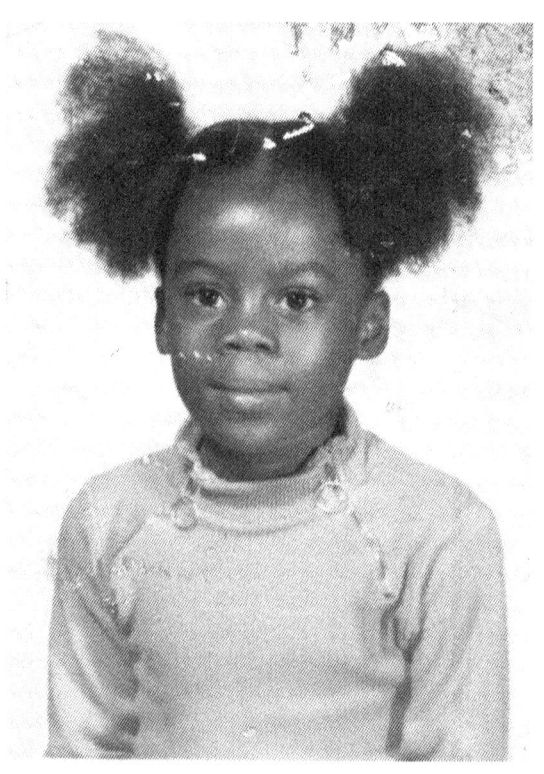

4. Taken in a New York elementary school, this photo shows Jeomie in a soft pastel pink shirt as a student. She is portraying her uniqueness through her hair design with her Afro puffs of two puff balls.

Phyllis East

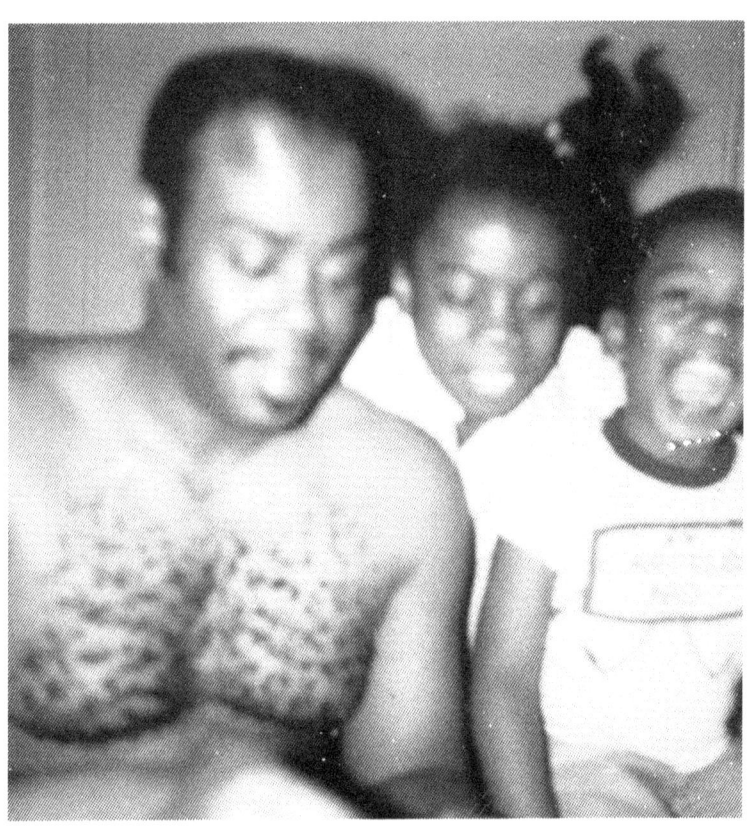

5. Loving her father very much, this photo shows Jeomie at 8 years old in between her father and her brother Robert.

Phyllis East

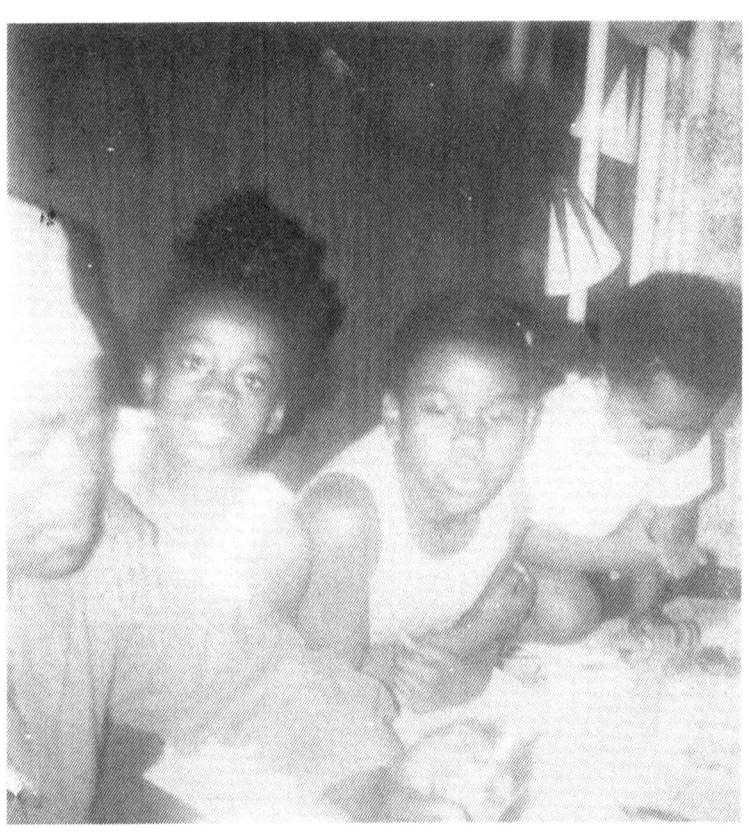

6. A joyous birthday party for her brother
Robert, Jeomie is 9 years old, and situated
next to her brother who is surprised when
Weomie blew out his birthday candles.

Phyllis East

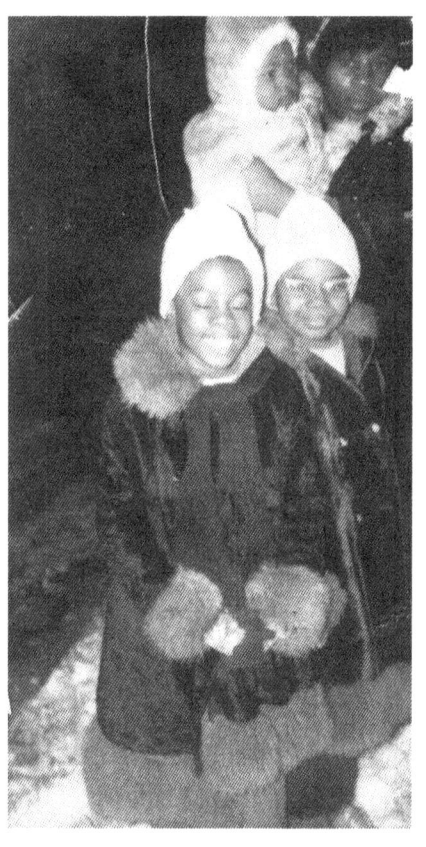

7. The cold weather has not kept either Jeomie, 9 years old nor her mother, sister, and brother from enjoying New York on a snowy day.

Phyllis East

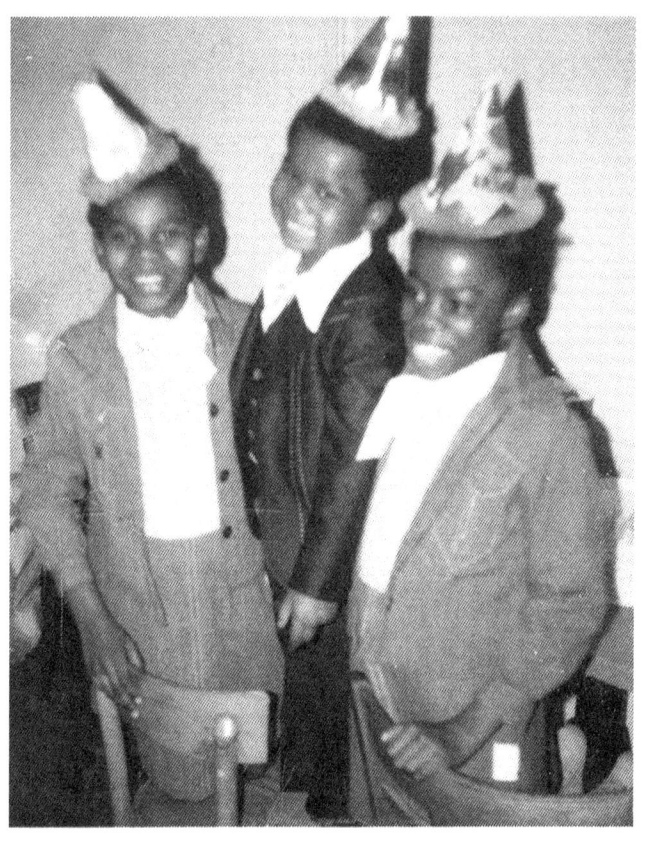

8. Friends and party hats help celebrate brother Robert's 5th birthday. Jeomie is 11 years in this photo, with Jeomie standing on the left.

Phyllis East

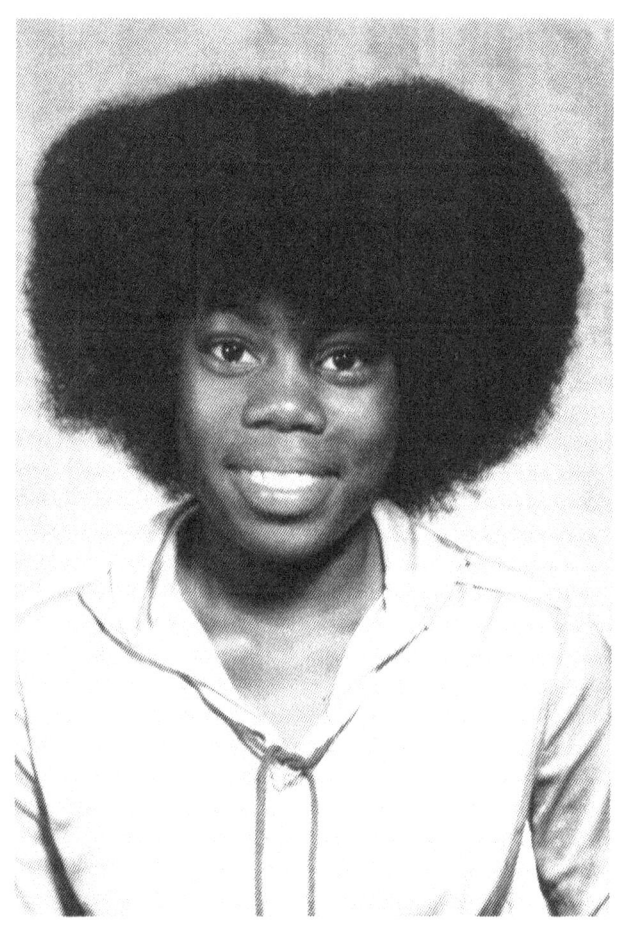

9. A extraordinary smile shows Jeomie bright and cheerful at 14 years old in her high school photo.

Phyllis East

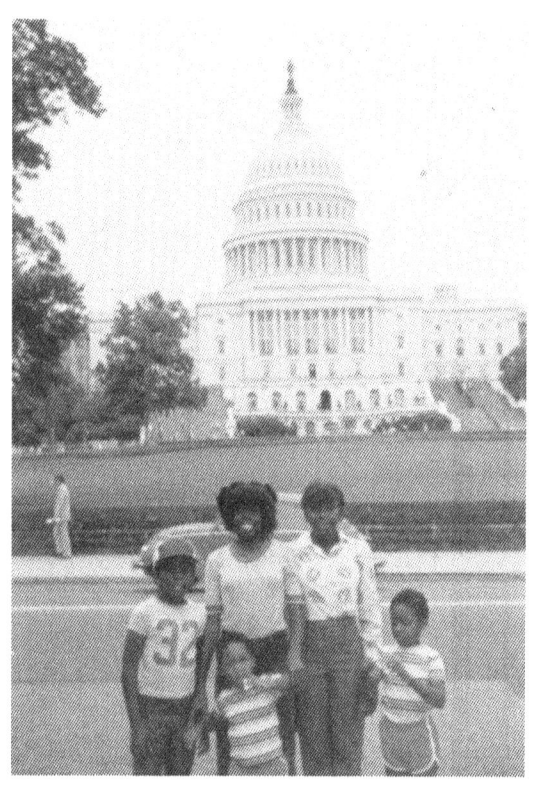

10. Washington DC was the place to visit for Jeomie when she was 16 years old. Two cousins in twin outfits stand with Robert and Weomie in front of the nations capitol building.

Phyllis East

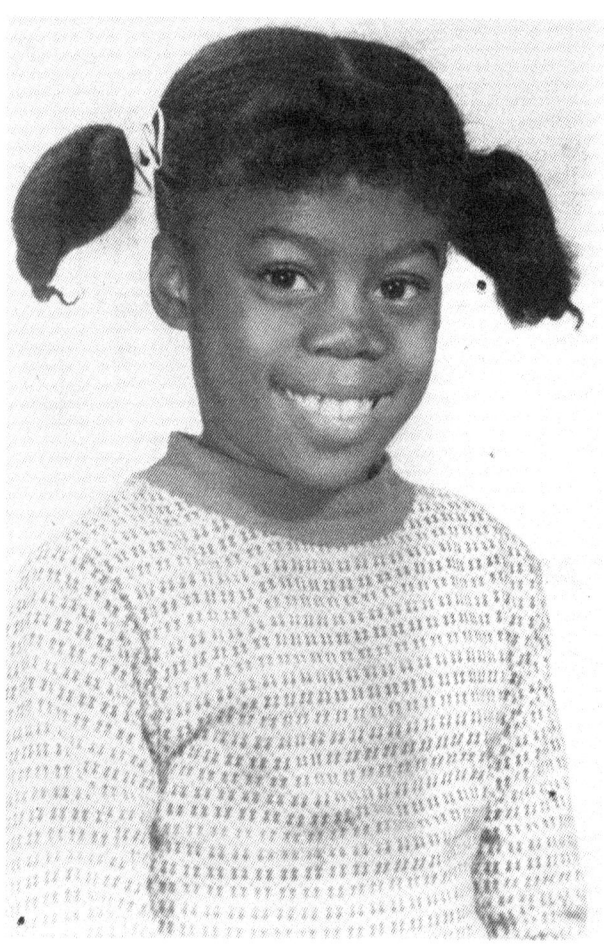

11. Jeomie appears to just love learning as she sits for her school photo.

Phyllis East

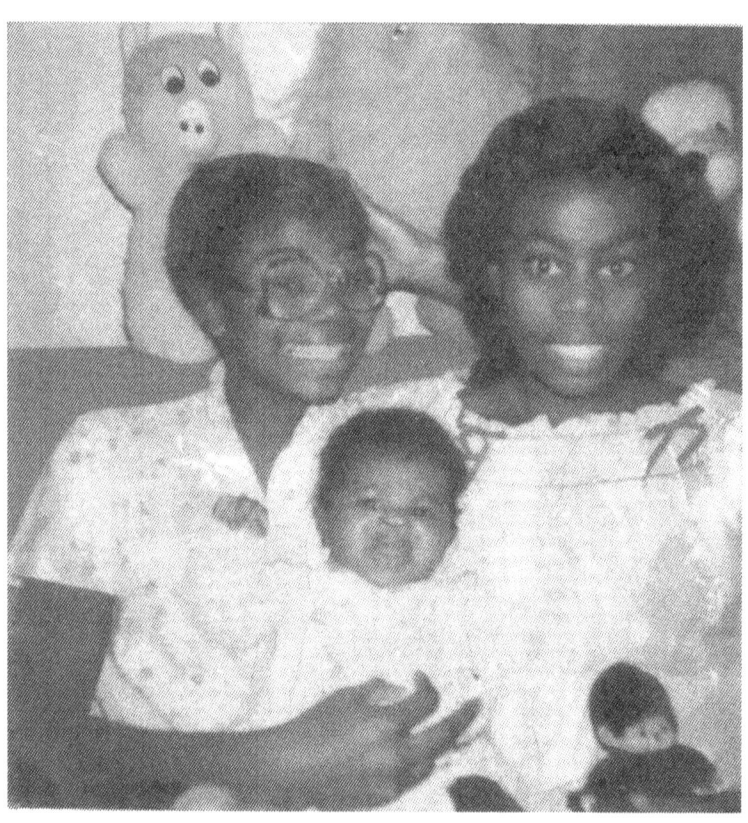

12. The three sisters, Weomie, Neomie, and Jeomie, are beautifully portrayed together in their living room at home with their stuffed animals.

Phyllis East

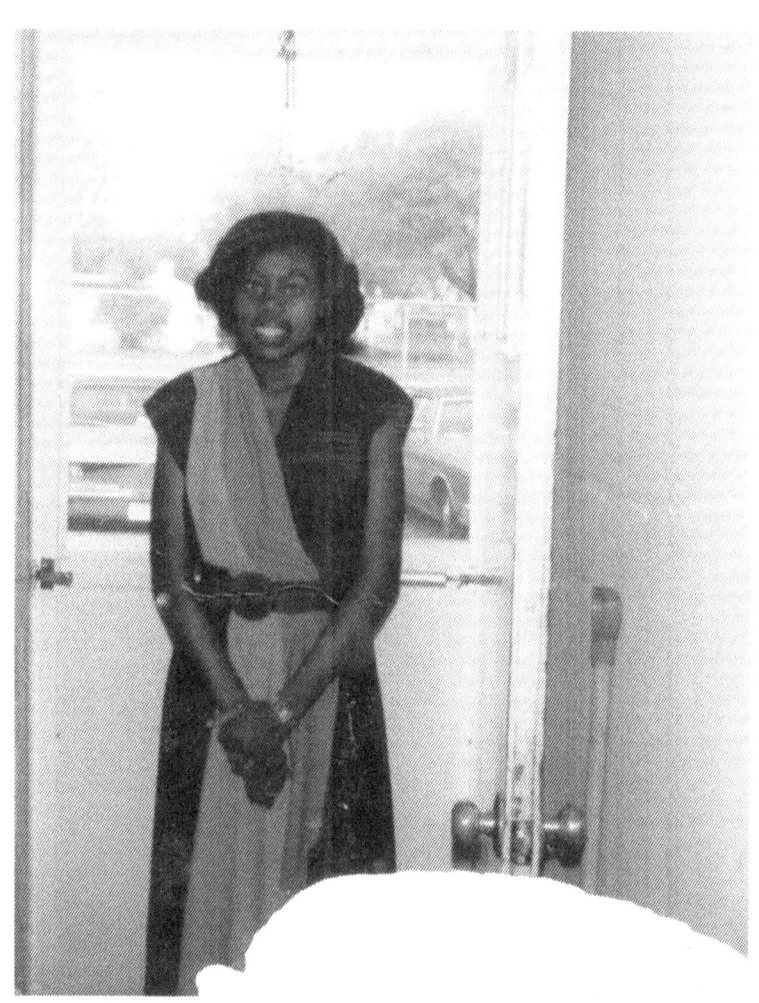

Phyllis East

The Early Life of Jeomie East
Struggling with Sickle Cell Anemia

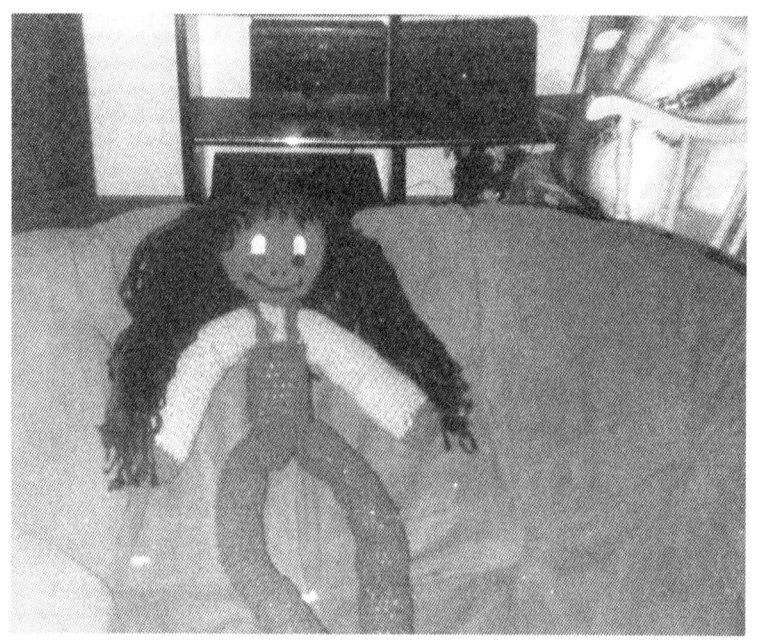

Phyllis East

A closing comment is necessary on Jeomie East's courage toward her illness which caused her much suffering. Jeomie kept meticulous notes on her medication. She had devised a system noted by colors and numbers to organize when it was necessary to take her medications. In her list of medications, she stated that certain substances were to be taken once a day, designated by a blue box. Other medications were to be taken several times a day, which was marked with a green box. A few of the medications were labeled with a red "x" to distinguish that if that particular medication was missed, the results could be dangerous.

This was quite an achievement for a teenager who was so ill.

About the Author

I would like to introduce myself. My name is Phyllis East. I am a widow and have been for the past fifteen years. I am also a Christian. I work hard in the church faithfully. I am in the choir and in the missionary circle. One of the things that I admire about myself is that I am a people person. I am a Nursing Assistant full-time. I went to college to become a licensed manager cosmetologist. Bowling and fishing are my favorite hobbies. I am a down-to-earth person.